▼ ▼ ▼ ▼ ▼ ▼ ▼ ▼ ▼ ▼ ▼ ▼

110 Mistakes
Working Women Make
and How to
Avoid Them

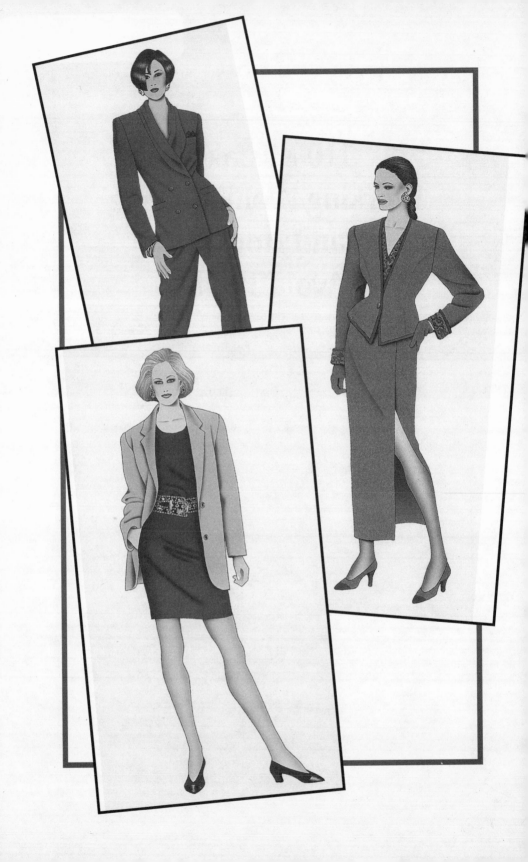

▼ ▼ ▼ ▼ ▼ ▼ ▼ ▼ ▼ ▼ ▼ ▼

110 Mistakes Working Women Make and How to Avoid Them

Dressing Smart in the '90s

JoAnna Nicholson

Impact Publications

Manassas Park, Virginia

Impact Publications
9104-N Manassas Drive
Manassas Park, VA 22111
(703) 361-7300

Library of Congress Cataloging-in Publication Data

Nicholson, JoAnna
    110 mistakes working women make and how to avoid
them : dressing smart in the '90s / JoAnna Nicholson.
        p. cm.
    Includes index.
    ISBN 1-57023-014-5 : $9.95
    1. Clothing and dress. 2. Beauty, personal. 3. Women
executives. I. Title. II. Title: One hundred ten mistakes
working women make and how to avoid them.
TT507. N46   1995
646'.34–dc20   94-31928
                                        CIP

Text and cover design by Joyce C. Weston

▼ ▼ ▼ ▼ ▼ ▼ ▼ ▼ ▼ ▼ ▼ ▼

SPECIAL APPRECIATION

To the much accomplished Renee Benton for her continuing loyalty, honest, flexibility, great knowledge, and incredibly fine work. And, for proving that Grandmothers can look super everyday!

To my sisters, Jane and Daphne, and my niece, Shannon, for believing in me and for using the principles I teach (coupled with their excellent taste) to prove everyday that looking great is a *lifestyle* worth accomplishing!

To the elegant and well-dressed Phyl and Ceci for their continuous unconditional support, great editing talents, wonderful ideas, and miraculously shared mischief!

To Caryl Krannich for making this book happen, for being the perfect role model for what it teaches and for being a terrific editor.

To Mimi, Trina, Rusty, Mary Frances, Shu Shu, Ruthy, Helen, Dorothy, Mia, Allison, Susan, Georgia, Annie, Bonnie, and Audrey for all of their loving support, trust, and friendship.

To all of the Color 1 Associates throughout the world especially Elizabeth Hermann, Sachi Matsumoto, Kathleen Spike, Maggie Quinn, Lea Hamilton, Kate Frost, Denise Schwartz, Janna Beatty, and Rebecca Page for their on-going conviction and work in showing clients how to change the way the world looks at them.

To #1 for his discerning awareness of the effort and results—it's mutual.

▼ ▼ ▼ ▼ ▼ ▼ ▼ ▼ ▼ ▼ ▼ ▼

Introduction

Who made the rule that you need to look "less than fabulous" in order to accomplish your work in an exceptional way? It's the '90s and *finally* we can give ourselves permission to break all of the old rules on how to dress for business except two:

1. *Always* look elegant and well-groomed. Depending on where you work, you may dress in classic elegance, casual elegance, trendy elegance, high-fashion elegance, feminine elegance or conservative elegance. And,

2. I want you to "Dress Smart" — that means playing by any reasonable rules your workplace or industry has (written or understood) until you get to the top, at which time you get to set the standard.

Elegant, accomplished working women come in all shapes, sizes, and ages. They may be poor, rich, or somewhere in between. They may be quiet, outgoing, or both, depending on the circumstances. And although they may spend a lot, or a very little, on their clothes they do have one thing in common and that is that they all have *developed* an elegant look!

If your industry or workplace has a written or understood "dress code," create a look for yourself that is even more stunning, yet *businesslike*, than the code suggests. Look totally elegant everyday and avoid creating any visual barrier

▼　▼　▼　▼　▼　▼　▼　▼　▼　▼　▼　▼

that may keep you from reaching your career goals. Wearing clothing that is viewed as "appropriate" for your workplace gives the impression that you are competent and a team player.

Dress equal to or better than the top female in your company. Think quality, not quantity. Strive for elegant simplicity, not overdone. To assure that you are *Dressing Smart in the '90s*, avoid making any of the following "mistakes" and use to your advantage the wealth of information in this book to support and expedite your personal career goals.

1

Ineffective Packaging
Fear of Showing Your Best Side

Heaven forbid that you might turn heads when you walk into a meeting — what's this world coming to? Will the meeting accomplish less? I suppose that there are those who feel that it would be better (more businesslike) if you looked forgettable instead of stunning. I would call those persons near-sighted or, perhaps, jealous. If more women looked great all of the time, the only "distraction" would be a woman who didn't! Men (and women) would be only too happy to "get used to" women who look fabulous all the time.

If you are fearful that you will look "overdone" and that people will be gazing at you with raised eyebrows instead of admiration, keep your look totally understated, yet elegant.

Low Returns on Your Investment
Having a Wardrobe That Doesn't Work for You

When you shop do you just fatten your closet? Most women really only utilize about 25% of their wardrobe in any given season. They buy things (a lot of them) that they have *never* worn, or have worn only once or twice. How many garments do you have hanging in your closet that still have the tags on them and they have been hanging there for several months?

Learn how to build a Smart Working Wardrobe that you can count on, that you feel *great* in, everyday! Understanding how to overcome mistakes #1 through #110 will empower you to look great all the time.

▼ ▼ ▼ ▼ ▼ 　3　 **▼ ▼ ▼ ▼ ▼**

Looking As if You Work in the Mailroom
Instead of the Boardroom
Not Having Any Million Dollar Looks

You can ask a room full of women to list their million dollar looks (outfits they already own that they feel, and look, like a million dollars in) and only two or three women out of fifty can write anything at all on their list.

Stop buying! Don't buy anything at all — unless it is equal to or better than the best look you have right now. Be able to look in the mirror and say, "Yes, I look and feel like a million dollars." If you can't say it, leave it — you will find something perfect the next time you go shopping!

Million dollar looks have nothing to do with the amount of money you spend on your clothing but they do have to do with "investment" — *a lifetime investment* because your future will be brighter based on the way you look right now!

4

Unfortunate Contract
No Sense of Style

M ake a contract with yourself and live up to it. As with any contract, the "small print" often contains vital data that you must read and understand in order to get the results you're wishing for.

This is the first time in history that women in their 40s and 50s look *better* — more stylish, more elegant and more "put-together" than women in their 20s and 30s. Mothers and grandmothers look more attractive than their daughters!

All of the "small print" in this book will assist you in developing a look uniquely your own — for *your* career! Why is developing a sense of style so important? Aside from the benefits of a tremendous boost in self-assurance, people automatically admire and project positive qualities and values onto individuals that are stylish in their dress.

▼ ▼ ▼ ▼ ▼ ▼ ▼ ▼ ▼ ▼

Looking Like You're Still Living in the Recession – The One Before Last

Old Fashioned

Wearing the old "dress for success" look touted by John Molloy makes you look out of date. Some women used to want to dress like all of their peers – to blend in, was to be safe. Now, many women want to standout as individuals, feminine individuals, but still look appropriate and professional.

You can look appropriate without looking prim, severe, boring or mannish.

Short-Term Profits Versus Long-Term Goals
Viewing Yourself in a Small, Rather Than a Full-Length Mirror

No one can dress well without a full-length mirror. Place it where you can walk a few paces away from it. Turn around fast. If your eye goes to the color or pattern you are wearing it is probably too bright, too bold and/or too large for you, causing you to look overdone or garish — certainly not a successful look.

If your glance reveals an overall "washed-out" or dull look, the color or pattern is more than likely too muted, too weak and/or too small for you. This is not a successful look!

If your eye goes straight to your belt, necklace or earrings, for example, the accessory may not be right for you and/or your outfit.

Learn to use your mirror to your advantage and let it help educate you. Check your stocking color. Is your shoe too heavy looking? Are your colors balanced and coordinated looking. Do they really enhance you? Does your hair style make the statement you want? Do you love the way you look from head to toe?

Lack of Strategic Planning
Misunderstanding the Difference Between Classic, Fashionable and Trendy

How are the top level women in your industry expected to dress — totally classic, more fashionable or trendy? "Classics" have a long life expectancy. "Fashions" have a medium life expectancy. And, "trends or fads" have a short life expectancy. Not classic: anything oversized, overstated or extreme (like big collars and oversized lapels); platforms; *very* short skirts; very wide pants, etc.

Classic clothing is never really out of style. How "fashionable" classically styled clothing appears is almost always dependent on the way you choose to combine classic garments and how current fashion is using or showing these items.

A current fashion does not go out of style as quickly as a trend. Note, however, that a fashion can become a "classic" and a fad can become a fashionable look if they hang around long enough. And, the fad that becomes a fashion can even become a classic if it stays around for a very long time.

For example, a shawl collar is classic, although it is moved to and from the forefront of fashion from time to time, while oversized collars are not considered classic because they are only "fashionable looking" once every decade or two. Vests are classic garments that are sometimes "in fashion" and are sometimes even given a trendy look — like when they are covered with buttons, lace and flowers.

▼ ▼ ▼ ▼ ▼   ▼ ▼ ▼ ▼ ▼

Unbridled Pioneering
Wearing Things That Look Like
They Belong at a Party

The boundaries between day and evening wear have been totally blurred — therefore we get to break all of the old rules, right? Yes, with the two exceptions written on the first page of this book. Review them if necessary.

Most women appropriately attired for their workplace will avoid: sheer, see-through fabrics; showing cleavage; *very* short skirts, anything that is too bare; and garments that are too glitzy.

▼ ▼ ▼ ▼ ▼ ▼ ▼ ▼ ▼ ▼

Misreading Your Market
Inappropriate Clothing for Your Workplace

Not all "fashionable" garments are appropriate for every workplace, of course. Stirrup pants, as of this writing, are an example of a garment that is considered classic only on the ski slopes and in riding circles. And although stirrup pants started as a trend, they are now considered fashionable and are being worn by women of all ages. Even though they are fashionable, they are not considered to be business attire unless you can wear a more sporty look to work. Stirrup pants were designed to be worn with boots rather than "flats" or "heels" — the "stirrup" of the pants is *not* supposed to be seen.

Before you invest in any garment or accessory, ask yourself if it will serve you well in your workplace and help you create the exact look you want. If the answer is yes, and the item is trendy, ask yourself another question: are you willing to spend your money on something that you may not be able to wear more than one season?

If you are on a budget make your first purchases "basic," classics. Besides being classic in style, what makes a garment basic? The following: a solid color; all stitching matches the garment color exactly; the buttons are the same color as the garment; there are no details like epaulets or contrasting trim or braid — in other words, perfectly plain and simple. (Do not read boring.)

10

Acquisition of Quantity Instead of Quality

Don't do it. Get out of the habit. If "it" is equal to or better than the best look you have right now, go ahead and buy it. Otherwise, you are just fattening your closet as you shop. It is far better to wear the same *perfect* outfit once or twice a week than have three or four outfits that are not as great on you!

Profile
Looking Dowdy

Caused by any one, or innumerable mistakes listed in this book. Avoid making these mistakes and you are guaranteed to look super every day! Women who look dowdy in the '90s may be viewed as being behind-the-times — not a positive business image.

Noncompliance With Code
Looking Too Casual

If the garment or overall look of your outfit is too casual or inappropriate for *your* workplace, you are making a visual statement that you don't know what's appropriate and/or that you don't care.

Examples of styles and garments that look out-of-place in some businesses, but are appropriate in others, are jeans; garments with fringe; "ski" sweaters and stirrup pants. While none of these are appropriate in a bank or law firm, they are each appropriate in some place of business: a designer wearing jeans with a beautiful jacket; an assistant editor of a fashion magazine wearing a suede fringed jacket with a matching skirt; a saleswoman of outdoor clothing or sporting equipment in a ski sweater; a travel agent in stirrup pants with a matching jacket.

▼ ▼ ▼ ▼ ▼ | 13 | ▼ ▼ ▼ ▼ ▼

Profile
Sloppy Looking

A sloppy appearance, created by poorly put-together, ill-fitting, unwashed, unironed, mismatched, or stretched-out clothing, also sends the message that you don't care how you look and/or you don't know how to dress. All in all, that you are *not* confident or competent in "at least one" aspect of your life — casting doubt on your competence in other areas.

Lack of Synergism
Buying Separates That Never Make an Outfit

Two of the reasons why most women only wear about 25% of their wardrobe is that they continually buy separates that either cannot be combined to create an outfit or that they do not know how to combine.

To solve the first, get in the habit of buying entire outfits — that doesn't mean that you must buy all of the pieces that were made to go together, although, that's (usually) a nice easy way to look coordinated, but not as original as some of you may like. However you may feel about this, please, always buy a matching top to any skirt or trousers (or look for a matching top made by *anybody* right away). You will never be sorry that you have this "base," as it is the *easiest* way to look coordinated and elegant.

Learning how to combine separates to create great looking outfits is fun, and not really that difficult — like learning a new "trick" in word processing that will make your life easier forever. (Review #28, #29 and #30.) An easy way to have a pulled together look is "to bring the bottom color up." This simple feat can pull together separates that you would never believe could be combined into unique and great looking outfits.

The minute you buy a "bottom" (skirt, trousers, etc.) start looking for a neck accessory (necklace, scarf) that matches it. Then immediately start putting this principle into use by combining the new bottom and neck accessory with tops and jackets that are already hanging in your closet.

No Competitive Edge
Falling Behind the Times — Wearing an Out-of-Date Wardrobe

A woman is not born with the innate talent to beautifully dress herself, her significant other and her children. She needs lessons.

It's like typing. Everyone can type (just like we can all get dressed in something everyday). Without lessons, you hunt and peck — I call it "hit or miss." With a couple of lessons you may be able to type 17 words a minute with 3 errors. With more lessons, you get faster and more accurate. After lessons, if typing is part of your life, you just get better and better at it.

If you stop typing, you can get "rusty" — and, besides, new equipment is developed and you may not know how to use it skillfully (new styles of shoes, textured stockings, pants in all widths and lengths, skirts in all shapes and lengths, belts that would have dazzled Cinderella, etc.)! HELP? Keep reading this book, but also subscribe to at least one fashion magazine that will help you keep up with the newest elements *and* how to combine them. For specialized assistance call (800) 523-8496 to find the most highly trained image consultant — a Color 1 Associate — closest to you.

Misinterpreting Your Value Line
Wearing Garments That Are Unflattering
to Your Body

You can create any look and wear any style you wish as long as you get the scale, fit, and balance right for your size and shape.

Yes, very short women and very tall women can look great in long jackets and short jackets, long skirts and short skirts, as can very thin women and very full figured women.

If you have allowed your size and shape to be a limitation to you in the past, it's because you've been bombarded with less than accurate advice and a mind set of old myths and you've not had the knowledge to challenge these myths. In reality, no matter what you look like you may do most everything all other women can do. Did I say most? There are always a few exceptions. For example, most women with very heavy legs won't be wearing very short skirts, but they can wear short skirts. Think about it for a second. If only women with perfect legs wore short skirts, very few short skirts would ever be worn.

In Need of Restructuring
Badly Tailored Garments

Fit is *so* important to creating a great look! Expensive garments will look less expensive if they fit poorly and less expensive garments can look *very* expensive (if the fabric is good) when they are tailored to fit *you.*

Make friends with a good tailor/dressmaker and spend the money to get the fit right. If you shop quality instead of quantity, you will probably be able to afford this extra expense. If not, *never ever* buy anything that doesn't fit right to begin with.

A Cut Below
Skirts That Are Shaped Wrong

Slim fitting skirts (straight skirts), no matter what their length, should taper inward (become slimmer) at the hemline to give you a fashionable, sleek appearance. Sometimes referred to as "pegging" your skirt, the taper starts just below the widest part of your hips and slims gradually to the hem. Unpegged skirts can make you look pear-shaped and dowdy. Avoid longer "A" line skirts that fall below the knee and dirndl skirt styles — they can make any body shape look dowdy.

Cutting It Too Close
Clothing That Is Too Tight

If it's "too" tight, especially across your bustline or your bottom it won't look elegant. You must judge, or ask an elegant friend to help you judge, if the garment simply looks classy and feminine (and maybe just a touch sexy) or if it's too sexy for *your* workplace or just plain sleazy.

▼ ▼ ▼ ▼ ▼ | **20** | ▼ ▼ ▼ ▼ ▼

Cramping Your Style
Jackets That Are Too Tight Across Your Seat

Yes, it is definitely a fit problem, but it is such a prevalent mistake that it deserves its own number. Check the view of your backside every time you check your front. For a little extra ease, move your buttons over if you can. If you can't, wear the jacket open (if it looks good open). Clothes that fit too tight can make a person look larger or less elegant.

▼ ▼ ▼ ▼ ▼   ▼ ▼ ▼ ▼ ▼

Using Faulty Substitutes
Wearing A Too-Casual, or Stretched-Out,
Cardigan as a Jacket

A cardigan is a terrific option to a jacket if it looks elegant. Judge it this way: if it looks equally as smashing as your best jacket, wear it to work!

22

When Too Much Is Too Much
Wearing Your Sleeves Too Long

Too long sleeves give the impression that you are wearing "hand-me-downs" or that you do not know what size you wear. Do you need a petite size only in blouses and jackets? Sleeves with ruffles that "are supposed" to hang down over your hand are fine *if* they go with your total look, and you assure me that you won't ask your company for disability if they get caught in a machine.

Creating a Deficit
Sleeves That Are Too Short

I f you feel elegant when you push-up or roll-up your sleeves, do this with any garment you already own that has this problem. Do you need a tall size in blouses and jackets? It often works to buy blouses and jackets a size or two larger than you would normally need (make certain the shoulder still fits well) then have the garment taken in if necessary.

Selling Yourself Short
Wearing High-Water Trousers

"High-water" pants are men's most prevalent mistake. They do not look better on women. Here are some general guidelines: the wider the trousers, the longer they should be (not more than 1 inch off the floor in the back *with your shoes on*). Classic width and slimmer straight legged trousers should end *no higher* than the place where the heel of the shoe meets the main body of the shoe. More slim cut trousers that taper toward the ankle are worn a little shorter (because if they are slimmer around the ankle they won't be able to come down over the shoe that far) but they should definitely cover the ankle bone. A slight break in the front of your trousers is always nice.

Using Depreciated Assets
Garments and Accessories in Need of Repair

Wearing a garment or accessory that needs to be repaired ruins your look – don't do it. Train yourself to immediately repair or have repaired anything that needs it.

Looking Like Common Stock
Instead of Preferred Stock
Wearing Colors That Are Too Bright or Too Muted

If you are one of the approximately 50% of women who wear bright, vibrant colors well, wear them (and your best neutrals) exclusively! The other half of you are more enhanced by colors that are more subdued or muted; wear them (and your best neutrals) exclusively!

If a color is too vibrant for your coloring it can make you look garish. If it is too toned-down/subdued for your coloring it can gray or sallow your skin and make you look washed-out. Get your brightness level and your colors just right for you so *you* can look successful and stunning all the time.

▼ ▼ ▼ ▼ ▼   ▼ ▼ ▼ ▼ ▼

Cut-Rate Colors
Wearing Colors That Are Not Flattering

You *can* wear every color and look great if you know *your* best shades, your best red, for example, versus mine. There are many shades of every color. For instance, green: lime, celery, kelly, mint, emerald, sea, apple, etc. I am most enhanced by emerald green while all other greens turn my skintone sallow or gray looking. Do you know what your *best* green is? Your *best* blue? Your *best* purples?

If you are not certain what colors and color combinations flatter you most, check the Resource Section. I do not recommend any of the "seasonal" or "cool/warm" types of color theories as it is my experience that at least 50% of the colors in their packets are not enhancing to the individual.

Did you know that some "consultants" who *do* color charts have had only 2 to 3 hours of color training (because the remainder of their 2-day training is on how to sell you makeup)? The Color 1 Associates that I recommend have studied approximately 4 weeks before their actual technical training which lasts *6 full days*. The Associates are also on a lengthy apprenticeship program after their training. They paid $2,895 plus airfare, hotel and food expenses for their training versus the $150 some other companies charge for their 2-day *makeup sales training*.

Ill-Fated Mergers and Acquisitions
Unsuccessful Color Combinations

If you love to wear the "fashion" or "in" colors of the season even though they may not be enhancing to you, try using an accent of one of your best colors next to your face.

Contrary to popular belief, *all* colors can be successfully worn in *any* place of business. And they can all be mixed — it's how you combine them *and* the balance you achieve that makes the difference between looking well put together or like you don't have a clue. Look to your own unique coloring for your best clue!

If your coloring is delicate looking, lighten up darker colors and dark, or stronger, color combinations. For example, a navy suit worn with a red blouse is "lightened-up" by gold buttons as is a black and brown tweed jacket that is worn with a black or brown skirt. A gold necklace (a tiny chain is not enough) also adds lightness. Wear earrings that are a combination of one of the dark colors and gold.

If your coloring is stronger, gutsier looking, it may not be necessary for you to lighten stronger color combinations.

▼ ▼ ▼ ▼ ▼ ▼ ▼ ▼ ▼ ▼

Niche Marketing
Wearing Black and White or Navy and White Together and Thinking You Look Chic – Only Half of You Look Great

That means that 50% of you don't look great in these high-contrast color combinations. Everyone can wear black (in some way), navy and white. But *not* everyone can wear black and white or navy and white *together*.

Use your mirror to determine if you're flattered or over-powered by this high-contrast. If *you* look radiant, great! However, if your eye goes first to the color combination you will know that your outfit will enter a room before you do. You will look pale or washed-out by comparison. Instead of using white with black or navy, substitute your best light beige (a light version of your skintone) – creating a slightly softer contrast and a much more stunning entrance!

▼   ▼   ▼   ▼   ▼ $\boxed{30}$ ▼   ▼   ▼   ▼   ▼

Creating Lower Standards
Uncoordinated or Unbalanced Color Combinations

To make certain that your look is coordinated, or visually balanced, bring a touch of the "bottom" color "up." An ivory skirt worn with a blue blouse is *balanced* looking as soon as you add pearls or an ivory colored scarf. It is also perfectly balanced, of course, if you add an ivory jacket – BUT, if you take the jacket off, you need the ivory-toned neck accessory to look beautifully coordinated.

Other ways to bring the bottom color up: belt in the same color as the shoe; scarf or necklace the same color as the belt; and blouse or sweater the same color as the skirt or trousers. A jacket, vest or cardigan only count *if* you are certain that you'll leave it on.

Earrings are usually not large enough to act as a balancer. Avoid jumping the color from your shoes all the way to your neck or ear (i.e., red shoes and red necklace or earring with nothing red in between).

Wearing colors that have like value can create a well coor-dinated, balanced appearance. Combine: a light color with another light color (like pastel yellow with pastel coral); a medium color with another medium color (like medium turquoise with a medium purple); or a dark color with another dark color (like dark gray with dark raspberry). Delicate col-oring needs to lighten dark clothing combinations, and strong coloring needs to accent light combinations with a dark or bright color.

▼ ▼ ▼ ▼ ▼   ▼ ▼ ▼ ▼ ▼

Risky Business
Wearing Unfavorable Pattern Sizes

I f a pattern size is too small for you, it can make you look totally insignificant (the opposite of powerful); if a pattern size is too large for you, it can totally overpower you. Don't be afraid of prints, just learn which ones flatter you!

Everyone can wear medium sized patterns but not everyone looks great in small patterns or large patterns (with a few exceptions). Enhancing pattern size has nothing to do with your height or weight, it has to do with your coloring. Yes, I know it sounds goofy, and is contradictory to what you have learned, but it's true!

If your coloring is more delicate looking, wear small and medium sized patterns (or *very* lightweight, delicate looking larger patterns). Those of you who have stronger looking coloring (not having anything to do with your personality or body shape or size) and look best in more toned-down colors, look great in small and medium sized patterns and very blended looking large patterns. However, if your coloring is strong looking and you wear clear, vibrant looking colors well, medium and large patterns look wonderful on you (small patterns that have extremely high contrast, like black and white may be used if you will accent them with a bright color).

▼ ▼ ▼ ▼ ▼ 32 ▼ ▼ ▼ ▼ ▼

The White-Out Factor
Wearing Blouses That Are "Too" White

What? As strange as it may seem, only 50% of you are flattered by *pure* white — in a blouse or any other garment or accessory. Everyone can wear a white, soft white, and cream, but there is a major difference in how the various whites look on you.

If pure white tends to "jump off your skin" and look visually too bright or inexpensive on you, wear a softer white, off-white and cream. Avoid brownish and grayish looking whites; and unless your skintone is golden, avoid yellowish looking whites.

▼ ▼ ▼ ▼ ▼ ▼ ▼ ▼ ▼ ▼

Using Out-of-Date Technology
Wearing Your Makeup Like You Did When You Were in School

Wearing your makeup like you did in high school or college almost always makes you look older and uncontemporary. If you just got out of school you will want to develop a "polished" career look. Women were not born with the skills to apply makeup artistically, so they often look over-done or under-done. Find a person who can assist you in learning to apply flattering colors of makeup in a way that keeps your look contemporary. Don't trust everyone wielding a makeup brush to show you your best looks — sometimes makeup artists just teach you the "latest" (read trend) look when what you may want is simply beautiful, elegant makeup.

▼ ▼ ▼ ▼ ▼ ▼ ▼ ▼ ▼ ▼

Investments With Insufficient Returns
Spending Money On (and Wearing) the Wrong Makeup

- Makeup base too dark, too pink/peachy
- Too much makeup
- Too little makeup
- Too brownish blush
- Too reddish eyebrow pencil
- Over-plucked/too thin eyebrows
- Not "sketching" in missing eyebrows at outer edge
- Too much eyebrow pencil
- Putting blush on forehead, nose and chin
- Wearing too toned-down lip and blush color
- Wearing too bright lip color
- Wearing too much blush
- Wearing blush in the wrong place
- Not lining lips properly to create a beautifully shaped mouth
- Too brownish lip liner
- Applying eye shadow in the wrong colors and shape
- Not removing visible hair from upper lip and chin
- Too much eyeliner without being smudged

To learn more about career makeup application check the Resource Section in the back of the book.

"Just Don't Do It"

Wearing Athletic Shoes With Business Attire

Never! Don't do it! I won't even say please! No exceptions unless your doctor insists that no other shoe made for walking will work for your "problem" (have your problem fixed ASAP). American women are being laughed at all over the world because of this; and, if that's not enough to get you to stop doing it, most men would *never* consider a second look (at least not an admiring look) at a woman who is dressed this way — if you don't believe me, ask them.

Women all over the world have somehow managed to walk long distances without "sneakers" for centuries. Now, an American woman cannot seem to even go out for lunch, or to and from the parking garage, without putting them on.

Several companies make great shoes that are made for walking and standing that do not look like athletic shoes. You may not like their looks as well as the shoe you put on when you get to work, but, believe me, they will look one-thousand times better than wearing "sneakers" with your business attire.

Marching Out of Step
Shoes and Boots in Incompatible Colors

Somewhere along the way, women erroneously were taught that they could wear black shoes with anything. That's not correct now and it wasn't correct 30 years ago unless your hair is black or very dark brown. If you need an easy rule to follow, wear shoes and boots the same color as your hem (skirt, dress, trousers, etc.).

Another easy guideline is to wear shoes and boots in your hair color, lighter and darker versions of your hair color, and your skintone, depending on how light or dark your outfit is. For example, if you are wearing a teal suit, and you do not care to own, can't find or can't afford matching shoes, use your hair color — you will look *fabulously* coordinated.

Work to achieve a good "color balance" between your shoe or boot and your outfit by using a light or medium tone shoe with lighter colors; a light, medium or dark shoe with medium tone colors (depending on the look you want to create) and medium or dark shoes with darker colors.

If you look great in clear colors, shiny black patent leather will work for you. Those of you who are more enhanced by toned-down colors should avoid *solid* shiny black patent as the eye may be drawn to the "shine" at your feet. Patent in toned-down colors and neutrals other than black are fine as are shoes that are a mix of black patent and other materials such as leather, suede and canvas. Black patent in small strappy sandals will work as well.

A Match for Imelda But Still Not the Right Shoe

B esides having shoes in your hair color, and perhaps your skintone, you will want to eventually own shoes in any neutral you wear often and in your core colors. A core color is a favorite color that you wear a lot.

If you plan, and build, your wardrobe around two favorite neutrals and one or two favorite core colors, you can limit the number of pairs of shoes you need, allowing you more money (for the budget conscious) to buy better quality. A better quality shoe can upgrade an outfit; an inexpensive shoe can downgrade an outfit.

If you own both your favorite heel height and flats in your favored neutrals and your core colors, you will have the appropriate shoe for any outfit. The best "basic" (go with any-thing) shoes are cut low in the vamp and fairly low on the sides — giving you a longer legline and a less-heavy looking shoe.

The Old Foot-in-the-Mouth Routine
Inappropriate Shoes for Your Outfit

Wearing shoes that are too casual, the wrong style, or too visually heavy for the outfit are often seen mistakes. Make certain that your shoe or boot makes the same statement as your outfit — you may wear trendy shoes for work if you are wearing trendy clothing to work, but using a trendy shoe with classic clothing says that you don't know what's what. Using a casual looking shoe with a suit or a heavy looking loafer with a lightweight long skirt does the same.

Open strappy sandals are paired with sun dresses, evening dresses and lightweight casual clothing; therefore, they are generally worn during your free time unless your place of business calls for casual clothing.

Sling backs, or pumps with an open toe, are great for the workplace. No opaque stockings with these shoe styles or sandals, please. And when it looks, or feels, "wintery" outside, leave them in the closet.

Embellished shoes and boots (embroidered, studded, etc.) are wonderful if they go with the look you are creating to further your career. Jewels and other "sparkly" embellishments are usually worn by more trendy or high-fashion dressers.

Shoes and boots with heels covered in the same leather are dressier looking than those with heels that are stacked "wood."

Not Getting the Boot
Wearing Boots Incorrectly

Boots with long skirts are classic looking, while boots with short skirts are more trendy looking and come and go with fashion. Whichever you choose to wear, carefully select your stockings. An easy rule is to simply match the stockings to your boot or to your skirt. If your skirt does not cover the top of your boot, then the stockings should be opaque for all but the young or trendy. Use the same guidelines for boots worn with trousers.

▼ ▼ ▼ ▼ ▼ ▼ ▼ ▼ ▼ ▼

In Need of Being Well-Heeled
Shoes and Boots in Ill-Repair

No rundown heels, dirty or scuffed shoes or boots no matter what look you choose to create. They do not look smart, elegant or well-groomed.

▼ ▼ ▼ ▼ ▼ | 41 | ▼ ▼ ▼ ▼ ▼

Negative Contribution
Wrong Color Stockings

The color of your stockings can ruin an otherwise great look. On the other hand, if they are right, you won't notice them except as being part of your fabulous total look.

Never wear "suntan" looking stockings unless they are the *exact* color of your skin — which is very unlikely. They are often too dark and generally too "reddish" looking to have a natural appearance.

All women need a sheer skintone look with certain outfits. Slip one of your arms in the store's sample and hold it up next to your other arm. Your arms should match exactly.

When in doubt of what's best follow these guidelines: Wear your skintone or bone/ivory with *light colored clothing*. With *medium colored clothing* wear your skintone or bone/ivory if your shoe is medium in tone; your skintone or bone/ivory if your shoe is light; and your skintone, bone/ivory or a *very* sheer tint of the shoe color if the shoe is dark. With *dark colored clothing* wear a sheer tint of the dark shoe color; a skintone or a bone/ivory, depending on the look you'd like, the time of year, and the length of your skirt; or in the fall and the winter, an opaque stocking the color of the shoe (or possibly your hem).

Cyclical Declines
Stockings That Are Too Dark or Too Opaque

How sheer, medium-opaque or opaque you wear your stockings is dependent on the look you are creating for *your* place of business, how long your skirt is, the time of the year, and your age. "Age" is mentioned here because very short skirts teamed with very sheer stockings can look sleazy instead of sexy on "women of a certain age" — what age is that? You get to pick the number.

Opaque stockings work well with very long skirts and short skirts. A slightly opaque look is nice with a skirt that is just above the knee and a totally opaque look may be necessary with even shorter skirts in the fall and winter especially during the daytime.

Just slightly opaque stockings are great with skirts a few inches above the knee for both day and evening. Very thick stockings (almost as thick as a wool ribbed legging) are for trendy, funky looks.

Skirts that fall just below the knee cap need a stocking that is just a *sheer* tint of your neutral shoe color (navy, black, gray, etc.), bone/ivory or skintone. Avoid wearing opaque stockings with this length skirt. Generally speaking, in the late fall and winter, the shorter, or longer, your skirt gets, the darker you may wear your stockings. In the spring and summer months your stockings should be sheer tints of neutrals and colors, skintone and bone/ivory.

Avoid wearing opaque stockings in warm weather months.

Buyer Beware
Stockings That Are Too White

Avoid wearing stockings so "white" that you look like you should be in a nurse's uniform. Ivories/bones that are the least bit opaque can look too white or too "institutional." Check the color in natural daylight as well as in the same light you work in — lighting can really make colors change drastically and you do not need to start off your work day shocked to discover that your stocking color is not what you thought.

Buy Value, Not Market Trends
Stockings With Too Much Texture for Your Outfit

Stockings that have visible texture are definitely more appropriate with high fashion or trendy looks than they are with classic looks. Try them with long skirts and shoes or boots, or, for those who can dress really trendy at work, shorter skirts and shoes or boots. (Remember, within certain guidelines, the shorter the skirt the more opaque the stocking, even when they are textured.)

Small subtle patterns can be worn with more styles. Fish net and really open weave textures are not appropriate for *most* workplaces. "Swiss-dot" (sheer tint with matching dot) are more classic than other textures and can be worn with femininely styled suits and dresses. Try subtly textured stockings with pant suits – just a touch of texture or pattern showing at the ankle adds a lot of style.

The Minus Touch
Colored Stockings with Conservative Attire

Stockings in colors like blue, purple, red, etc., versus neutrals like black, gray, navy, bone, etc., come and go in fashion and are still "suspect" in several conservative business fields.

For the adventuresome who can wear colors to work, some great looks are created by: wearing a totally all one color look from shoe to earring (everything red, for example); putting together a monochromatic color scheme with lighter and darker tones of the same color, like mixing beige, camel, medium brown and dark brown, or light purple, medium purple and dark purple; and, definitely *not* for most work-places, by "color blocking" – using two or more blocks of colors like black shoes, red opaque stocking, short black skirt and a red top.

Multi-colored patterned stockings go to work only on the very trendy dressers.

Looking Like a Bag Lady
Stockings That Bag at the Ankle and/or Knee

Stockings that are too big for you, or that are *very* sheer, can "bag" at the ankles and knees. Try to find a size where your weight and height fall in the middle of the chart, not right on the edge where you are close to needing a smaller size or larger size. Having even a hint of lycra in your stockings helps keep them from bagging and helps them wear longer.

Creating a Lower Standard
Stockings with Runs, Holes and
Too Many Snags

K eep an extra pair of your most used neutrals at work. Change the minute you get a visible run or hole. Don't start the day with stockings that have several visible snags — save them to wear under trousers.

Taking Global Warming to An Extreme
Not Wearing Stockings When You Should

Not wearing stockings when it's hot outside isn't a mistake if you get to dress casually elegant at work. But if you are wearing an outfit that calls for stockings, put them on (working in air conditioning takes any excuse away).

How do you know if your outfit calls for stockings? If you are wearing pumps (even open toed pumps), sling backs, a suit, a pant suit, or a dress that isn't casual, wear stockings. Even many casual dresses look better with stockings. Also, if you are pretty much "all covered-up" (long sleeves, not much skin showing at the neck) bare legs look out of place.

If you don't want to have to wear stockings when it is hot outside, make *absolutely* certain that your work environment will allow you to wear the type of clothing that goes with a no stocking look. And keep your feet, toe nails, and legs beautifully groomed — no exceptions.

Tightening The Wrong Purse Strings
Uncoordinated Colors

If everything looks great but your purse, do you look great? NO! Carrying the wrong purse can ruin your look. In years past, our purse had to match our shoes and now both just have to go with our outfit. Actually, following the old rule is easy and "well pulled together looking."

A purse in your hair color is another great choice because it always goes with your color scheme – unless it is totally hidden by a hat, your hair color is part of every look you create.

Other excellent colors: your skintone (also always part of every color scheme you create), all neutrals you wear often and your core colors. Metallics are most often used for evening or for daytime casual, but can be used for daytime business if *your* business looks call for a metallic purse.

50

▼ ▼ ▼ ▼ ▼ ▼ ▼ ▼ ▼ ▼

Targeting The Wrong Market
Purses That Are the Wrong Style
for Your Outfit

A trendy or fashiony looking purse carried with classic clothing like a fringed suede pouch with a classic suit; a tailored, heavy looking leather shoulder bag used with a feminine elegant linen suit; or a delicate looking skin bag with a wool plaid suit are all examples of purse styles that aren't great with an outfit. Just as with everything else about your look (your hair, shoes, accessories) a purse must make the same statement as your outfit or you do not appear to know how to dress. Avoid doing anything that casts any "doubt" on any of your abilities.

Get in the good habit of emptying your purse into a lovely tray or basket at the end of each day (like a man empties his pockets). That will force you to reach for a purse that compliments your outfit the next day and fill it with only those things you need — an over-stuffed purse does not look elegant. Too much work? Then only wear outfits that look great with the one purse you want to carry everyday!

Falling Productivity
Using Purses That Look Inexpensive
or Ready to Fall Apart

No purses in need of repair, please. No "plastic" purses – you can buy quality leather goods on sale or at discount stores. Just as with shoes, a quality purse can upgrade your outfit; an inexpensive purse can downgrade it.

A purse without embellishment or any metal hardware showing is a great basic because it works beautifully with so many different outfits. Whether your other accessories and buttons are gold, silver or pearls, this purse will look good! If you lost all of your purses, this should be the first purse you buy. Always coordinate any metal color on a purse or tote with your jewelry, buttons and buckle. Please do not carry a bag that has gold hardware when you are wearing silver earrings, for example.

Playing on The Wrong Team
Unflattering Briefcases and Totes

Carry a briefcase or tote in your *most* used neutral or your hair color. If your hair is light, use a darker version of the same color — if you are a golden blond, for instance, use a golden camel or a light golden brown. If you can afford more than one briefcase or tote, add one in another neutral that you use a lot.

I recommend less "mannish" looking briefcases; also, buy the best quality you can afford. Please do not carry a large purse or tote at the same time you are carrying a briefcase unless you're headed for a plane or train. A smaller looking shoulder bag can be carried with a briefcase. Ideally, if you carry a small purse, it would fit inside your briefcase — in a "perfect" world.

▼ ▼ ▼ ▼ ▼ ▼ ▼ ▼ ▼ ▼

Ignoring Your Affiliates
Unmatched Luggage

It would be nice if they were, but your luggage does not have to be the same brand, or same style, but it should be the same color. Buy the best you can afford and stop using any luggage that looks like it won't make it through another trip — in other words, be proud to claim your luggage, not embarrassed.

▼ ▼ ▼ ▼ ▼ ▼ ▼ ▼ ▼

In Need of Retooling
Cheap Looking Pens

No cheap looking pens from other companies, banks, free giveaways, etc. A beautiful pen makes a nice statement about you. If you can't spend the money on one right now, use pens that are plain black, navy, or gray. When you acquire or are gifted with a beautiful pen, keep track of it.

▼ ▼ ▼ ▼ ▼ ▼ ▼ ▼ ▼ ▼

Tightening The Wrong Belt
The Improper Belt for Your Outfit

Embellished belts are fabulous with certain outfits. They can be worn to work if you get to work in clothing that calls for them. Remember, there are different types of embellishment, and each makes a different statement. Crystals on a belt are more "fashiony" than gold studs; and a Chanel style chain belt is far more classic than a belt that mixes leather, reptile skin, suede, crystals and studs.

Avoid wearing a trendy belt with a totally "classic" look. Very plain belts with just a simple but elegant buckle are basic and can be worn with many different looks (one and a half inches is a good width to begin with).

If you're wearing a belt on top of a printed garment, make certain that the color of the belt is *highly visible* in the print. Do a mirror check from a few paces away.

Getting Your Signals Crossed
Inaccurate Color Belt

Own basic and "statement" (if you love them) belts in the same colors as your most used neutrals and core colors, those that you have used for shoes and boots — this makes coordination rather easy.

Consider the metal color of your buckles. If navy is a basic neutral for you, and if you love both gold and silver jewelry, you will need two navy belts — one with a gold buckle and one with a silver buckle, unless you can find a navy belt with a covered navy buckle.

Take any metallic buttons into account when you put on a belt — gold buttons with gold belt buckles, silver with silver, brass with brass, and copper with copper.

Gridlock

Belts That Make a Different Statement Than Your Accessories

Make sure that your belt style and/or buckle style aren't "fighting with" the style of your outfit or any other accessory you are wearing: necklace, earrings, and buttons. An example of incompatibility is a contemporary rectangular shaped buckle worn with dainty filigreed round earrings.

Sometimes a stunning belt need be the only focal point of your outfit for the work place. Compliment this look with the selection of simple, but equally as beautiful earrings that make the same statement as your belt or, if your workplace allows, your earrings can be more dramatic.

58

▼ ▼ ▼ ▼ ▼   ▼ ▼ ▼ ▼ ▼

Ineffective Infrastructures
Inappropriately Attired Ears

Wear earrings that work from a style and color stand-point with your outfit. If your outfit is right for you at work, your earring will be as well. For example, conservative, classic clothing may be necessary in your place of business, so you wouldn't be wearing a glitzy or dangling earring to work anyway, because they do not make the same statement as your outfit.

Make certain that your earring style and shape is compatible with any buttons on your jacket or blouse. For example, a delicate pink and ivory cameo earring will not enhance a pink suit that has gold geometric buttons. Obviously, necklaces and earrings must work very well together, and with your outfit.

▼ ▼ ▼ ▼ ▼ ▼ ▼ ▼ ▼ ▼

Not Knowing Whether to Expand or to Down-Size
Wrong Size Earring

An earring that looks large on one woman will look medium sized on the next — it depends on your head size, of course, and your coloring. Yes, your coloring. If you have more delicate coloring, avoid *really* large earrings (unless they are very lightweight looking) because they can look "overdone" on you. On the other hand, if your coloring is stronger, small earrings can look insignificant.

Also, pay attention to your hair style. If you wear your hair back or if it's cut short, earrings are more necessary in achieving a finished, balanced look. Position clip earrings so that they rest right next to your face so they won't "flop" around when you move your head.

Missing The Mark
Earring Colors in Need of Auditing

Match metal colors — if your jacket buttons or belt buckle are gold, use gold at your ear; if silver, use silver. Metal colors can be mixed if the mix is carried out as a "color scheme." For example, if a necklace combines silver, gold and copper, the earring can be any one of those metals as can jacket buttons and belt buckle.

If your earring is a color, make certain that the *same* color is apparent in your outfit from a few paces away. This is especially important when working with tweeds, plaids, and prints where you may see a touch of that color up close, but from a few steps away it's not noticeable.

Being Cut Out of The Action

Necklaces That Are an Uncomplimentary
Shape for Your Neckline

Wearing a rounded necklace with a "v" shaped neckline, and using a necklace that hangs in a "v" shape with a rounded or jewel neckline are examples of necklaces that do not work well with a specific neckline. A good simple rule is to have the necklace follow the shape of the neckline.

Broadcasting the Wrong Signal
Necklaces That Are Too Ornate or Too Glitzy

If your place of business calls for clothing that may call for an ornate or glitzy necklace, then wearing one is not a mistake for you as long as you still look elegant. Glitzy and ornate necklaces are not part of conservative business attire, but if you love them and can't wear them at work, you can enjoy them in your free time.

If you need to dress more conservatively at work but still would really love to wear "more," try wearing a collection of simple or small necklaces, like several strands of pearls and gold chains together — add pearl and gold earrings. Or wear a larger pendant and keep your earrings simple. When in doubt under-accessorize.

▼ ▼ ▼ ▼ ▼ ▼ ▼ ▼ ▼ ▼

Chain Gang
Necklaces That Are Too Big or Too Small for You

If your coloring is delicate, avoid wearing a large necklace unless it is very lightweight looking. If your coloring is stronger, avoid small necklaces — they can look totally insignificant on you. One of the most common mistakes women make is wearing a small gold chain with everything.

▼ ▼ ▼ ▼ ▼ ▼ ▼ ▼ ▼ ▼

Getting A Busy Signal
Necklaces That Are a Disadvantageous Color

We have to deal with two types of "wrong color" here. The first is wearing a color that doesn't enhance your outfit. The second is wearing a color that doesn't enhance you!

To make certain the color of your necklace works well with your outfit, the color needs to be repeated at least once somewhere: in a print, the skirt color, the blouse color, or the belt color. Make sure that you can see the relationship of the colors from a few steps away.

If the colors in your outfit are great on you, the necklace color will be as well. Everyone can wear both gold and silver; if you look best in clear, vibrant colors, avoid wearing dull, tarnished metals. If you are more enhanced by toned-down, muted looking colors, avoid large amounts of bright shiny metals.

Troubles of Major or Minor Proportion
Necklaces That Are an Adverse Style or Design for Your Outfit

Avoid wearing a tailored gold necklace with a floral print; a rounded necklace with a geometric print; an ethnic necklace with a classic suit; or a trendy fashion-forward necklace with a conservative dress.

If you are not certain that an accessory is "additive," leave it off. Remember that your necklace and earrings must look great together and with your outfit. A common mistake is using a strand of pearls with "everything" — it's almost as if every mother once told every daughter that, "A strand of pearls is always appropriate." Maybe that was in the day that women of all ages wore sweater sets with pearl buttons — a great classic look with a strand of pearls.

Strategic Decisions
Misplaced Pins

Pins can be wonderful if you can figure out exactly *where* to place them, and, if they work in harmony with the style and shape of the garment you are pinning them on. Take into account any buttons, necklace and earrings. Examples to avoid: a square pin placed on a rounded or shawl collar (like shapes compliment); a pearl pin with gold buttons (a pearl and gold pin with gold buttons would be great); a delicate floral pin with a tailored chain choker (if the pin has a touch of gold in it, try hanging it on a more delicate chain or grouping of chains to give a pendant effect).

▼ ▼ ▼ ▼ ▼ ▼ ▼ ▼ ▼ ▼

Rattling Someone's Cage
Noisy Bracelets

B racelets that make noise can be an irritant or distraction to those you work with. So, if you don't work alone, no bracelet noise, please.

68

▼ ▼ ▼ ▼ ▼   ▼ ▼ ▼ ▼ ▼

Getting Cuffed
Bracelets That Make a Different
Statement Than Your Outfit

Three small bracelets worn together look more conservative than one bracelet that dangles or one large
embellished cuff. A lot of smaller bracelets stacked up the arm
look great with an outfit that calls for them, just as glitzy,
ethnic or other specifically styled bracelets may be worn with
outfits that they enhance — just make certain that the look you
are creating makes the statement that you wish to make at
your place of business.

Avoid wearing bracelets and rings that compete in style
and/or color with each other, your other accessories and your
buttons.

Being Out of Step With the Time
Wearing a Watch That Doesn't Compliment Your Outfit

The most common mistakes here are wearing a watch that is too sporty for your business attire; one that has a band in a color that doesn't go with your outfit or look good with your skintone; or, one that has gold on it when you are wearing silver jewelry or visa versa. Keep your watch in your purse if it isn't "additive" to your look.

In Need of Down-Sizing
Rings That Are Too Large

A ring (one only) that is quite large, or large looking on your hand, makes an unusual/dramatic statement. If wearing a large ring adds to a total look that is elegant and dramatic, yet appropriate for your place of work, great! If not, wear your larger rings in your free time. The same applies for trendy looking rings.

Excess Inventory
Too Many Rings

There are classy elegant men and women who feel that women who wear more than one ring on a hand have an inexpensive look. Others disagree. Does it look elegant, or "cheap?" My advice is that *less is more* but you must decide for yourself. And, should you decide to wear more than one, make absolutely certain that the rings compliment each other in style and color.

Quality Uncontrolled
Too Glitzy Buttons for Your Work Place

B uttons that have crystals, rhinestones or sequins are not appropriate for more conservative business attire. If the buttons on your jacket are keeping you from wearing it to work, or looking appropriate at work, you could change them. Otherwise, enjoy the jacket in your off hours.

Foreign Correspondence
*Wearing Scarves That Do Not
Match Your Outfit*

If you are wearing a green dress, for example, with a multicolored scarf, the scarf must have *visible* green it — the exact, shade of green. A tiny amount of the color in a pattern may not be enough to be seen from a few paces away — check it in your trusty mirror.

And, while you're looking in the mirror, check to make sure that you are not looking "engulfed" by your scarf. There are many ways to beautifully tie a scarf that will show just the right amount of scarf for you and your outfit. Check the Resource Section.

Faulty Analysis
Glasses That Are Shaped Incorrectly for Your Face

Avoid a double eyebrow look by selecting glasses that follow the shape of your eyebrows. Glasses that are too small for your face can make your eyes look closer together (sometimes even cross-eyed) — if you love smaller glasses and feel they give you an avant guard or "interesting" look, that's fine as long as you promise me that you look elegant in them.

Avoid glasses that "droop" down on the cheek, angling toward the jaw line — they can create a real "down-line" that can make you look tired and old!

Glasses that have fancy detailing across the bridge of the nose definitely draw attention to the nose area and can make your eyes look closer together as well as make your nose look big or "strangely" shaped. Real "fashiony-looking" glasses can limit your use of earrings and necklaces — if you wish to wear glasses that make a definite statement of their own, keep your earrings and necklaces very simple if your workplace is conservative.

▼ ▼ ▼ ▼ ▼   ▼ ▼ ▼ ▼ ▼

Looking at The World Through
Rose-Colored Glasses
Unenhancing Lens Colors

Avoid lenses that are tinted rosy, yellowish, bluish, greenish or any other color that gives you a bruised look under, and around, the eye.

Consider getting a reflective coating on your lens so your eyes aren't hidden behind "mirrors" that may be distracting to others.

Made in the Shade
Glasses Frames in Unflattering Colors

Metallics and frameless looks are more versatile than colors. If your skintone is golden, or your hair has golden highlights, your best metallic will be gold. Silver frames can work well with ivory skintones and platinum, ash blond, ash brown, silver or white hair colors. If you look best in toned-down colors select soft-toned metallics. If you look best in bright colors select a bright, shiny metallic. Ideally metallic frames should match any metallic accessories you are wearing.

Also, for those of you who would like a "frameless" look, consider those glasses that have a minimum amount of metal as support for your lenses.

Tortoise shell appears more casual than metallics and frameless looks but it is generally fine for daytime attire. Your most flattering tortoise will be a combination of your skintone and hair colors and works best when you are wearing your neutrals. Tortoise is not dressy enough to be worn with a "little silk dress or suit" out to dinner, or to cocktail parties, or black tie affairs. So if you are to only have one pair, avoid tortoise and colors. A plastic frame does not usually look elegant enough for all of your day and evening looks.

If you love frames in colors, select them from your core colors and only wear them when you are using that color in your outfit.

Skirting The Issues #1
Rising Hemlines

It's difficult to give strict directional advice as what looks short on one woman will look very short on another. Use the following as an approximate: Measure the distance from the top of the knee to the crotch. One-half of that measure (or shorter) above the knee is a very short skirt. One-fourth of that measure (or maybe an inch or two longer) above the knee is a short skirt. For example, if the measurement is 12", a very short skirt would be 6" (or more) above the knee and a short skirt would be 3" above the knee or less.

Look at your legs, decide how much of them you want to show. Look at the business you are in, decide if *really* short skirts fit with your career goals. Take a third look, decide if you look classy and elegant. Review the shoe, boot and stocking sections. If you look great in really short skirts but they are not appropriate for your workplace, look forward to wearing them for your non-business occasions.

Skirting The Issues #2
Dropping Hemlines

A couple of inches above the ankle bone is usually long enough for daytime attire. When a skirt comes all the way down around your ankles it can make you look like you're engulfed in fabric and living in another time. Use your mirror to help you decide – does your outfit look out of place for your place of business? Do you look elegant or enveloped?

If your skirt appears just a little too long, try wearing it with a sleek looking shoe with a heel or a boot with a heel to raise the hem, creating more inches between the bottom of the skirt and the floor. Now take another look. If it still looks too long it must be shortened – maybe only an inch!

▼ ▼ ▼ ▼ ▼   ▼ ▼ ▼ ▼ ▼

Skirting The Issues #3
Dowdy Lengths

There's sort of a "no man's land" for skirt lengths — aptly named because most men don't pay attention to women who wear their skirts this length. What is this often dowdy length? From just below the knee cap to 1 to 2 inches below the *bottom* of the calf — it depends on your height and your leg length. Two inches is a lot more on a woman who is 5' 1" than it is on a woman who is 5' 9".

Women of every height can look great in both long and short skirts — it's getting the skirt long enough or short enough, knowing what style top and/or jacket to combine the length with, and what stocking and shoe or boot style creates the perfect look for *you*.

If you wear your skirts hovering around your knee, wear *sheer* stockings and high slender heels or medium heel height shoes that are cut low in the vamp and low on the sides — other style shoes can give a dowdy look with this skirt length. It's nice to let the curve of your knee cap show.

80

▼ ▼ ▼ ▼ ▼ ▼ ▼ ▼ ▼

Unfounded Support System
The Wrong Underwear

How can someone other than an intimate other tell? By the bulges that show above and below your bra, panties and pantyhose. By the slip that shows in your kick pleat when you walk. By the "odd" shape of your bustline. By visible panty line. By the way you pull your panties down in the back when you don't think anyone is looking.

There are women in the underlovelies departments that have been trained to fit you in a bra — ask. Own slips in black and beige. Own short slips, semi-short slips and long slips if you wear clothing in several lengths. Buy slips that have a slit and line it up with the slit in your skirt (no slips showing in slits, please).

Most women need to buy their panties a size larger than they usually do to get them to fit properly — especially after they are washed. Try panties on (over your own) in the store. Sit down. Stand up. If they ride-up, don't buy them. If they make a visible panty line, they are too tight. Own both beautiful briefs and bikinis. Briefs (buy sexy styles with high cut legs) are sometimes handy to tuck your top into when you need an extra smooth line. Skintone briefs are great to camouflage a colored top so that it doesn't show through lighter skirts and trousers.

Always feel as good about your under-clothes as you do your over-clothes. No safety pins in bra straps, no holes in panties. Wear matched sets.

Taking The Wrong Position
Poorly Positioned Shoulder Pads or No Shoulder Pad When Necessary

Shoulder pads are great "balancers" for women's bottoms, helping create that desirable "v" shape — a shape that looks wider at the shoulderline than it does at the hipline. The opposite of this "v" shape is a pear shape which makes a person look dowdy.

Have women given up their shoulder pads? Not until men do — they give them the same flattering shape. Most of us have given up the huge padding and settled in on medium size to smaller pads depending on what we are wearing and the natural width of our shoulders. Some women with a natural shoulder width that is at least as wide as their hips can do without pads in some garments. They still need a little padding in garments that make their shoulders look sloped or narrow in comparison to their hipline.

If your shoulder pads are placed too close to your neck, they can give you an unflattering narrow shouldered look. Use your trusted mirror and note the placement of your pads. They should be situated so that they make your shoulderline look a bit wider than, or at least equal to, your hips.

▼ ▼ ▼ ▼ ▼ | 82 | ▼ ▼ ▼ ▼ ▼

Ignoring The Risk/Reward Ratio
Plunging Necklines

S how cleavage only during your free time.

Looking Like The Dog-Days of Summer
Bare Arms With Too Low-Cut Armholes

In hot summer months a woman may wear a sleeveless dress, jacket, or vest to work if the armhole is cut high enough so that you cannot get even a glimpse of her bra or her breast. If you work in a conservative field where there is still a written or understood rule against bare arms, play the "game" until you are the boss.

Easy Out
Too Clingy Knits

Knits are super for business wear for all body types as long as they are not too tight. Too clingy knits show bulges above and below your bra, and at the waist and hips. Some of the new "body slimming" slips, panties and stockings can help *smooth-out* this concern, as can camisoles and slips that help knit fabrics glide over the body instead of cling to it.

▼ ▼ ▼ ▼ ▼   ▼ ▼ ▼ ▼ ▼

Expanding Into The Wrong Territory
Garments and Fabrics That Do Not Retain
Their Configuration

Fabrics that bag and sag ruin the look of an otherwise great outfit. Avoid purchasing inexpensive rayons and inexpensive knits unless you are willing to give them up after one season. Wearing a slip will help them hold their shape, as will not wearing them to death. Before you buy, ask yourself if the garment will be a good investment that will help you achieve your career goals!

Market Myopia
Fabrics That Allow Investigation

S heer and "peak-a-boo" fabrics are not generally considered businesslike; well, maybe "monkey businesslike."
How sheer is "too sheer?" You get to judge. Does it work if you
wear a camisole under it? Only you know your place of business, its spoken and unspoken "codes," and your career goals.
When in doubt, save sheer fabrics for playtime.

Discounts
Materials That Are Too Informal

It depends on where you work, of course. Cotton knits are too casual if you work in a law firm, for example, but may be perfect if you work in the office of a veterinarian, or if you are a vet. When you try something on and you *feel* casual or sporty in it, do not wear it for business attire unless sporty/casual is the look you are striving for at work.

For the budget conscious, or those who like a sparse wardrobe, buy garments in fabrics that are considered wearable year-round in your climate. Consider: silks, including raw silks, tropical weight wools, good quality rayons and rayon files, quality polyesters and polyester files, microfibers, knits, and blends of synthetic and natural fibers.

Although silks are considered year-round fabrics, in those climates that have cold weather months, lighter weight silk dresses, skirts, and slacks are more approriately worn in the evening.

Blouses in fine cottons, linens, and silks of all weights are worn year-round both day and evening.

Gross Domestic Product
Oversized or Overextended Sweaters

They can look great with leggings, stirrup pants, and both long and short "skinny" skirts and full skirts. With pants, especially, they make a more fashiony and often more casual statement. With skirts, it depends on the fabrics and the over-all look as to whether you will look fashionable, trendy, casual or sloppy. You get to decide if these looks are a mistake for you in your work place. Note: a different state-ment is made by a sweater that hugs in under your bottom and one that hangs straight.

Selling Into The Wrong Market
Wearing Sweaters That Look Like They Belong
on the Ski Slope or at a Party

"Outdoorsy" looking sweaters and sweaters with lots of glitz are usually best kept for your free time unless you work in an environment where you know that they are expected attire.

This doesn't mean that those of you who work in more conservative fields cannot wear sweaters that are "embellished." There are some great sweaters that are embroidered or have pearls or studs that you may be able to wear to work. If you aren't certain, watch what the top women in your company are wearing and follow their lead until *you* get to be the leader.

Tip: If you want to make something embellished look more conservative, keep everything else you are wearing very simple and understated.

Mismanaging The Leading Edge
Wearing Conflicting Necklines

Wearing a notched collar blouse with a shawl collar jacket does both an injustice. The easiest rule is to have your blouse style repeat the same line as your jacket. If you would like a little more variety, here are a couple of tips: a jewel neckline, just slightly rounded neckline and "tank" style tops look fine with all jacket styles. A "v" neckline works well with notched collar lapels and collarless jackets that also have a "v" shape.

▼ ▼ ▼ ▼ ▼ ▼ ▼ ▼ ▼ ▼

Not Delivering The Goods
Not Knowing How to Merge Separates

Looking elegant and uniquely stylish isn't difficult once you know how. The easiest way to start to build a "smart" wardrobe is to keep your look uncomplicated and under-stated. Remember, quality, not quantity. Well tailored. Wonderful colors and color combinations for you.

Begin by creating a base — an all one color look in a skirt or trousers with a matching blouse or simple sweater. Your first base could be in your favorite neutral. You can change the look of your base, simply by what you choose to wear on top of it — a jacket, vest, tunic, duster, cardigan, belt, scarf, dif-ferent accessories — in any of your best colors.

Your second base could be in one of your core colors. Create different looks by wearing the bottom of one base with the top of the other (don't forget to bring the bottom color "up") and you'll have an excellent start on forming a great Smart Capsule Wardrobe. Use a variety of jacket and blouse styles — each will increase the individuality of your look. To learn more about how to create a Smart Capsule Wardrobe, see the Resource Section in the back of the book.

Modus Operandi
Not Profiting From Your Individuality

Add individuality to your new Smart Capsule looks by taking a currently fashionable item and using it in your own unique ways. Let's take the vest as an example: you can wear it without any thing under it (if the arm hole is cut high enough); over numerous styles of blouses (make sure the necklines work together) including a sleeveless blouse or shell/tank; over a tunic; T-shirt; sweater; another vest; with a scarf; necklace (one strand or many); embellished with a pin (one or several); under a jacket in place of a blouse or over a blouse; and over a jacket.

The vest could be lace, silk, velvet, satin, wool, rayon, etc.; jewel encrusted or studded (depending on your workplace); it can be plain or patterned; have "statement" buttons, plain buttons, or no buttons; it can have lapels in all shapes, or no lapels at all; it can have any style neckline from a mandarin collar to a deep "v"; and, it can be worn over any style or length skirt, trousers, jeans or shorts.

Add uniqueness through your accessory use: Wear no jewelry one day and a lot the next; maybe you *always* wear a great belt and you have put together your Smart Capsule to showcase your belts — making a "signature statement." Perhaps *your* signature statement is always wearing a necklace. If so, the blouse and jacket necklines in your Smart Capsule must be perfectly selected to work with your necklaces.

Statute of Limitation
Wearing a Dress That Is Not Equal in "Stature" to a Suit

Why is it that we see so few good dresses in the work place? One of the reasons is that there are so few good styles to choose from. Another is that many women seem to select dresses with a different part of their brain — the part that still wants to be a little girl, at a party, or living in another decade. A dress that makes a statement equal to that of your best suit doesn't have to have a jacket but it does have to have all of the same wonderful qualities of that suit: it is a style that is perfect for *your* workplace; fits you well; has good quality fabric and construction (doesn't bag or sag after a few wearings); it's a great color on you; you've accessorized it perfectly; and, you *love* it and are willing to wear it very often.

It's been said that a dress has to be *very* tailored looking to match the "authority" of a suit, but it really only has to be elegant and appropriate (remember, equal to or better than the best look you have right now).

Dresses that come with matching or coordinating jackets are super, as are dresses that are styled so that you can wear one of your existing jackets over them. If you like a lot of variety, look for a simple (do not read boring) dress with beautiful lines that you can accessorize with different belts, scarves, or jewelry.

The Imperfect Coverup
Wearing the Wrong Coat or Jacket

Are you making a negative "arrival and departure" statement? When you take your coat off, are people surprised at what you are wearing underneath? Coats need to make a good impression because they are often your first impression or your last impression, and sometimes your only impression.

Select coats in styles and colors that go with your clothing styles and colors – your most used neutrals and core colors. What's your weather like? The more "basic" the coat, the more things you can wear it over. Make certain that a long coat is long enough to cover your longest skirt and that all of your coats and jackets fit with ease over suit jackets.

Choose the style carefully. If you tend to dress more feminine elegant, do not purchase a coat that is trendy looking, made out of a sporty fabric, is severely tailored, has sporty stitching or sporty detailing, etc. If you love long, fuller skirts, do not buy an extremely straight coat, but one that has a bit of fullness. You get the picture – make sure that everyone looking at you gets a pretty one.

▼ ▼ ▼ ▼ ▼ ▼ ▼ ▼ ▼ ▼

Myth Versus Reality
Sacrificing Comfort for Looks

It's being done everyday — particularly in shoes — lovely to look at but uncomfortable to work in (they were *so* pretty — on sale, too — and you just couldn't live without them and they didn't have your "exact" size). Skirts and trousers that are "just a touch" tight in the waist can annoy you all day as can bras that dig into your skin, and trousers that are too high in the rise.

Garments like these start getting left at home, making you feel guilty because you wasted your money on them.

▼ ▼ ▼ ▼ ▼ | 96 | ▼ ▼ ▼ ▼ ▼

Inefficient Integration
Sacrificing Looks for Comfort

Comfortable, grubby, baggy and sloppy are not synonyms. Comfort can be found in any style and shape so it's never necessary to make this sacrifice. When you try something on, sit down in it, walk around in it, and ask yourself how it *feels* on your body. Confining? Scratchy? Uncomfortably tight when you sit?

Follow one of the best smart wardrobing rules in the world – don't buy it unless it is equal in looks and comfort to the best look you have right now!

Polluted Hair

Dirty or uncombed hair is not appropriate in any business situation.

98

Unexplored Opportunity
Disorganized and Disorderly Hair

Too many women get "all dressed up" to go to work and their hair ruins their image. Tips: If you are wearing your hair like you did when you were in high school or college, the style is more than likely no longer as enhancing and contemporary looking as it could be. Always check the back of your head for "hair-holes" — I believe that's a southern term. The back of you is as important as the front because if someone sees the back of you first, they may never be interested in finding out what the front is like.

A great hair cut is only as good as you can make it look on a daily basis. If you do not have the time or talent it takes to keep up a certain style get one that you can manage — *but* make sure that your hair *looks* great all of the time.

Find someone who can cut and style well — consistently. If he/she is not consistent, *change* your allegiance. A good hair cut may cost as little as $10 to $15 — a good "design" for *you* may (but not necessarily) cost more. But once it's shaped beautifully you will be able to have it maintained by anyone who cuts and styles well. (Show your stylist your new design within the first week you've had it done.)

▼ ▼ ▼ ▼ ▼ **99** ▼ ▼ ▼ ▼ ▼

Looking As If You Just Dyed
Unbecoming Hair Color

There's just an awful lot of hair out there that is too ashy or too brassy looking. If your hair is brassy looking it can sallow your skin and/or give you an inexpensive appearance. If it is too ash, it can gray and dull your skin, causing you to look washed-out.

Your hair color is critical to your image and if the color is wrong it can really diminish your beauty, even if everything else is perfect. Find a good colorist (not necessarily the same person that cuts or styles your hair).

▼ ▼ ▼ ▼ ▼   ▼ ▼ ▼ ▼ ▼

In Need of Damage Control
Damaged Hair

I f your hair looks damaged, it damages your appearance!
Get your hair trimmed and then vow to keep your hair in
good condition.

Too Bossy a Fragrance

It's neither businesslike nor sexy. A person should be able to discern another's fragrance *only* when in *very* close proximity. Use your fragrance sparingly and ask an honest friend or coworker if they can tell when you've entered the room.

▼ ▼ ▼ ▼ ▼   ▼ ▼ ▼ ▼ ▼

Banned
Chewing Gum

Don't. Unless you are alone and not on the phone. It looks unprofessional and inelegant and can be distracting and a major irritant to others.

▼ ▼ ▼ ▼ ▼ ▼ ▼ ▼ ▼

Traveling Third Class
The Way You Look When You Travel

How proud do you feel about telling your seatmate on the plane or train what you do when they ask the inevitable question? Could they guess what you do by the way you are dressed? Would they guess executive, mid-level, entry-level, or unemployed?

What impression are you giving others about yourself and your company when you travel? Would they want to do business with your company based on the way you look? Yes, you do reflect on your company's reputation, as well as your own, every time you get dressed — whether you are going around the world, or just to the mail box.

Travel stylishly and comfortably (remember, comfort and sloppy are not synonyms). Select your outfit according to your arrival activities and pretend that your seatmate may be the prince you've been waiting for or the chairman of your company. If you are headed straight for a meeting, *or* are being met by a business associate, dress for business (unless you are traveling overseas in which case you may want to travel more casually — read elegant casual — and change into your business attire before you arrive). See my comments on luggage — #53.

Reality Check
Perceiving Yourself Differently
Than Others Do

It's very difficult to look at yourself objectively — it's almost as if you become immune to yourself. If you feel that your same old favorite lipstick and hair style looks great, or the same style clothing you've gravitated to for eons is great on you, or you don't receive compliments on a regular basis and/or you lament that you continue to attract the same type of men (those that you'd rather not), it's definitely time to change your image!

Your friends and family may not be your best resource for objectivity because they are "used" to you. Change can be unnerving because the "old" you has a certain familiarity and comfortableness. As you begin to look "different" (read "better") heads turns — when you first realize that someone turned to look, you may wonder if your slip is showing! Get used to admiring glances.

When you are attempting to change the way you look, avoid shopping with a friend that says, "that doesn't look like you" when you ask her/his opinion — it's not the old you that you're shopping for.

▼ ▼ ▼ ▼ ▼ **109** ▼ ▼ ▼ ▼ ▼

Taking Too Long of a Power Nap
Not Paying Attention to Details

A great look is attained, in part, by paying attention to all of the "little" details. (See #1 through #110.) Here's an abbreviated check list — it's *assumed* that your look is perfect for your career goals:

Hair:	Stylish.
Makeup:	Perfect (neither too much nor too little).
Earrings:	Right statement and color with your outfit; right size/shape for your face & coloring.
Necklace:	Right statement, color and size; works with your earrings and with the shape of your jacket/blouse neckline.
Necklines:	Compatible jacket and blouse.
Shoulder line:	A tiny bit wider than (or at least equal to) your hipline.
Color:	Great shade for you.
Clarity:	Not too bright; not too toned-down.
Color Combination:	Not too strong/overpowering; not too weak/washed-out looking.
Outfit:	Well put together, totally elegant million dollar look.
Fit:	Perfectly tailored for you.
Stocking:	Perfect color, texture and fit.
Shoe:	Perfect style, color, and condition.
Purse:	Perfect shape, style, color, and condition.
Coat:	Same statement; compatible color; long enough.

▼ ▼ ▼ ▼ ▼ ▼ ▼ ▼ ▼ ▼

Undervaluing Your Current Investments
Looking Inelegant

There is no excuse for not looking your best *all* the time! If you look great and feel great about the way you look, it will bring you incredible success in your career. An additional unexpected and fabulous bonus is the positive radiating effect you have on everyone whose life you touch and on people whose lives they touch – your boss and coworkers and their families; everyone you talk with on the phone and those they interact with; your significant other and his boss; your children and the people in their lives (friends, teachers, family, coworkers)…all because you feel terrific about the way you look!

▼ ▼ ▼ ▼ ▼ ▼ ▼ ▼ ▼ ▼ ▼ ▼

RESOURCE SECTION

POLISH YOUR IMAGE WITH
A NEW CAREER MAKEUP LOOK

Career 1™ Makeup was designed to give you the sophistication and polish you deserve to assist you in looking both successful *and* beautiful *every day!* What makes Career 1™ Makeup different from other makeup?

It's all in the special colors! Career 1™ Makeup is a division of Color 1 Associates, Inc., International Image and Style Consultants, whose clients include Ambassadors, Senators, Cabinet Secretaries, presidents of major international companies, movie stars, top models and even Miss America.

If Barbara Walters used makeup colors that look stunning on Connie Chung, she would not look her professional best and vice versa. If Oprah were to use makeup colors that look great on Toni Braxton, she would not look "smart", and vice versa.

The "secret" to your most terrific career look is to select the Career 1™ Makeup Kits that contain those colors that were specifically designed to give your unique coloring an incredibly polished and well put together appearance.

RICHLY MUTED
(toned-down medium to dark colors)

Select this kit if your coloring more closely resembles that of Kathie Lee Gifford, Whitney Houston, Barbara Walters, Wynonna, Oprah, Nancy Reagan, Cindy Crawford, Julia Roberts, Whoopi

▼　▼　▼　▼　▼　▼　▼　▼　▼　▼　▼　▼　▼

Goldberg, Diane von Furstenberg, or Barbra Streisand. If you would also like to achieve a more quietly subtle look for certain occasions, you may wish to add the Elegantly Gentle Kit to your "makeup wardrobe."

ELEGANTLY GENTLE
(toned-down medium to light colors)

Select this kit if your coloring more closely resembles that of Candice Bergen, Linda Evans, Phylicia Rashad, Jane Seymour, Cicely Tyson, Betty Ford, Jane Pauley, Glenn Close, Meryl Streep, Cybill Shepherd, Mia Farrow, Shelley Long, or Faye Dunaway. If you would also like to achieve a more dramatic, yet still subtle, look for certain occasions, you may wish to add the Richly Muted Kit to your "makeup wardrobe."

STRIKINGLY CONTRAST
(bright medium to dark colors)

Select this kit if your coloring more closely resembles that of Elizabeth Taylor, Connie Chung, Diahann Carroll, Cher, Kimberly Aiken, Jacqueline Kennedy Onassis, Barbara Bush, Queen Elizabeth, Ruth Bader Ginsburg, Connie Selecca, Toni Braxton, Delta Burke, Kate Jackson, or Jaclyn Smith. If you would also like to achieve a lighter, more delicate, look for certain occasions, you may wish to add the Beautifully Light & Bright Kit to your "makeup wardrobe."

BEAUTIFULLY LIGHT & BRIGHT
(bright medium to light colors)

Select this kit if your coloring more closely resembles that of Marilyn Monroe, Dolly Parton, Diana Ross, Princess Di, Hillary Clinton,

▼ ▼ ▼ ▼ ▼ ▼ ▼ ▼ ▼ ▼ ▼ ▼ ▼

Melanie Griffith, Janet Jackson, Sally Jessie Raphael, Kristi Yamaguchi, Sandra Day O'Connor, Ivana Trump, Tyra Banks, or Mary Hart. If you would also like to achieve a more dramatic look for certain occasions, you may wish to add the Strikingly Contrast Kit to your "makeup wardrobe."

These products are all full size, not sample size; so with the exception of your lipsticks, the products should last you at least a year.

To compliment your Career 1™ Makeup Kits, JoAnna has available *Career 1™ Skin Care* – Exceptional products of superior quality at conservative prices. To order, call (800) 523-8496.

CLASSES, SEMINARS, AND WORKSHOPS

JoAnna Nicholson personally offers classes, workshops, and seminars on total image enhancement subjects for every career. To arrange one for your company, your organization, or for just you and your friends, call (800) 523-8496.

A sampling of program topics available:

How to dress when your job depends on it and your firm is
    depending on you
Creating contemporary business looks with classic clothing
The art of feminine business dressing
The corporate makeup look: subtle and effective
Using accessories appropriately to finish and polish your look
Stylish business dressing on a limited budget
How to shop like an expert
Taking the guess work out of what makeup colors to wear
    with what

▼ ▼ ▼ ▼ ▼ ▼ ▼ ▼ ▼ ▼ ▼ ▼ ▼

Mastering the look of luxury

Anti-aging wardrobe, makeup, and hair style tips

Basic or advanced wardrobing for women: a popular and necessary training for women of all levels

Exploding the myths: the navy suit/white shirt "dress for success look" actually weakens the appearance of more than half of all women

Creating illusion: looking great no matter what your shape or size

Tying one on: how to tie scarves that add a professional and subtle touch of flair

Style: how to get it…how to keep it!

Professional and pretty on the run: wardrobing and makeup tips for busy women

Wardrobe auditing: how to plan, coordinate, utilize, and organize your existing wardrobe for maximum effectiveness

Appropriate sexy business dressing

Or, let JoAnna design a program especially for you!

For the best advice available anywhere on your most enhancing colors, Joanna recommends Color 1 Associates, located throughout the world. Associates offer Personal Color Charting consultations and related image services to assist you in discovering how to look great *all day, every day!* Call (800) 523-8496 for the Associate nearest you.

Create a Smart Capsule Wardrobe – for a "How To" booklet, call (800) 523-8496.

Available soon in your local bookstore, *How to Be Sexy Without Looking Sleazy,* by JoAnna Nicholson, Impact Publications, 1995.

114

INDEX

▼ ▼ ▼ ▼ ▼ ▼ ▼ ▼ ▼ ▼ ▼ ▼ ▼

CAREER RESOURCES

Contact Impact Publications to receive a free copy of their latest comprehensive and annotated catalog of career resources (books, subscriptions, training programs, videos, audiocassettes, software, and CD-ROM).

The following career resources are available directly from Impact Publications. Complete the following form or list the titles, include postage (see formula at the end), enclose payment, and send your order along with your name and address to:

IMPACT PUBLICATIONS
9104-N Manassas Drive
Manassas Park, VA 22111
Tel. 703/361-7300 or Fax 703/335-9486

Orders from individuals must be prepaid by check, moneyorder, Visa or MasterCard number. We accept telephone and FAX orders with a Visa or MasterCard number.

Qty.	TITLES	PRICE	TOTAL
___	60 Seconds and You're Hired	$9.95	_____
___	110 Mistakes Working Women Make and How to Avoid Them: Dressing Smart in the '90s	$9.95	_____
___	Almanac of International Jobs and Careers	$19.95	_____
___	Best Impressions in Hospitality	$14.95	_____
___	Best Jobs for the 1990s and Into the 21st Century	$12.95	_____
___	Change Your Job, Change Your Life	$14.95	_____
___	Complete Guide to Public Employment	$19.95	_____

▼ ▼ ▼ ▼ ▼ ▼ ▼ ▼ ▼ ▼ ▼ ▼ ▼

Qty.	TITLES	PRICE	TOTAL
___	Complete Guide to International Jobs & Careers	$13.95	_____
___	Complete Job Finder's Guide to the 90s	$13.95	_____
___	Directory of Federal Jobs and Employers	$21.95	_____
___	Discover the Best Jobs for You	$11.95	_____
___	Dynamite Answers to Interview Questions	$11.95	_____
___	Dynamite Cover Letters	$11.95	_____
___	Dynamite Salary Negotiation	$13.95	_____
___	Dynamite Tele-Search	$11.95	_____
___	Educator's Guide to Alternative Jobs & Careers	$14.95	_____
___	Electronic Resumes for the New Job Market	$11.95	_____
___	Find a Federal Job Fast!	$12.95	_____
___	Five Secrets to Finding a Job	$12.95	_____
___	From Army Green to Corporate Gray	$15.95	_____
___	From Navy Blue to Corporate Gray	$17.95	_____
___	Graduating to the 9-5 World	$11.95	_____
___	Great Connections	$11.95	_____
___	Guide to Careers in World Affairs	$14.95	_____
___	High Impact Resumes and Letters	$14.95	_____
___	How to Be Sexy Without Looking Sleazy	$6.95	_____
___	How to Get Interviews From Classified Job Ads	$14.95	_____
___	How to Succeed Without a Career Path	$13.95	_____
___	Interview for Success	$13.95	_____
___	Job Search Letters That Get Results	$15.95	_____
___	Jobs & Careers With Nonprofit Organizations	$15.95	_____
___	Jobs for People Who Love Travel	$12.95	_____
___	Jobs in Russia and the Newly Independent States	$15.95	_____
___	Jobs in Washington, DC	$11.95	_____
___	Jobs Worldwide	$15.95	_____

▼　▼　▼　▼　▼　▼　▼　▼　▼　▼　▼　▼

Qty.	TITLES	PRICE	TOTAL
___	Mistakes Men Make That Women Hate:		
	101 Image Tips for Men	$6.95	_____
___	New Network Your Way to Job and Career		
	Success	$12.95	_____
___	New Relocating Spouse's Guide to Employment	$14.95	_____
___	Red Socks Don't Work! (men)	$14.95	_____
___	Resumes for Re-Entry: A Woman's Handbook	$10.95	_____

SUBTOTAL _____

Virginia residents add 4.5% sales tax

_____

POSTAGE/HANDLING ($4.00 first title
and $1.00 for each additional book)　　4.00

Number of additional titles x $1.00

_____

TOTAL ENCLOSED _____

NAME_____

ADDRESS_____

_____

❑ I enclose check/moneyorder for $_____ made payable
to IMPACT PUBLICATIONS.

❑ Please charge $_____ to my credit card.

Card # _____ Expiration date: ___/___

Signature_____